CW00409619

Good Housekeeping

home
spa
treatments

Rosie Mills

series editor
Vicci Bentley

HarperCollins*Illustrated*

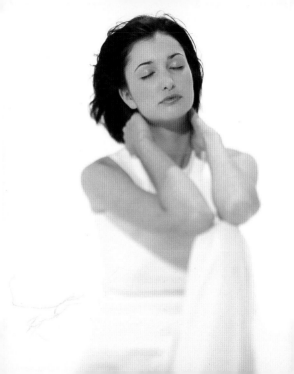

contents

Sparkling fresh sensations in ice-cool waters that purify, recharge and rebalance? Warm, soothing soaks that send waves of relaxation flowing through your body?

Water therapy is actually one of the oldest forms of healthcare. The early physicians of Rome, Greece and India were quick to realise the healing potential of natural springs. The Romans built baths near medicinal springs and wells. The Greeks practised the ancient art of aromatherapy by putting oils in water. Later, as spa towns (named after Spa in Belgium, the original centre) cropped up all over Europe, drinking of and bathing in the healing waters became a popular pilgrimage in the eighteenth and nineteenth centuries.

Today, spas are much more than health resorts offering only pure water therapy. These oases of calm incorporate the latest holistic treatments for mind and body harmony. Essential oil and herbal therapies, stress-relieving exercises like yoga and t'ai chi, healthy detoxifying diets – they are all now part of the spa experience. Taking time out to truly relax and invigorate yourself from the inside out is probably one of the wisest health investments you'll ever make. The trouble is, when is there the time, or money – or both – for you to be able to visit a spa?

Mindful of the fact that today most of us seem to live our lives on the run, this book has been specially created for you and your hectic schedule. A realistic spa programme that's not only easy and cheap for you to follow in the comfort of your own home – but also a spa programme that will take up only one day of your time. A day that's totally different from any other. Starting to relax already? Good. Because relaxing is one of the most effective ways of counteracting stress.

With a variety of water-based treatments such as hydrotherapy and thalassotherapy, pampering aromatherap baths, relaxing massages, simple yet effective yogic breathing and stretching, quick energy-boosting juices and healthy, cleansing menus, you can unwind, recharge, soothe and rebalance a jaded mind, body and spirit. If you're one of the lucky ones with a weekend to spare, indulge to the hilt. Only a few hours? Select a treatment or two. *Home Spa Treatments* has been devised to give you a realistic blueprint for healthy spa living. making it easier to adapt to your lifestyle, and leaving you feeling full of vitality on the inside, beautifully glowing on the outside.

hydrotherapy ('hydro' from the ancient Greek word meaning water) is one of the most refreshing ways to treat every part of you.

hydro

herapy

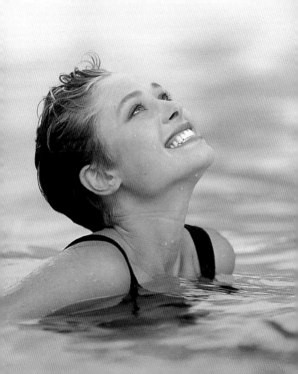

the
therapeutic
value of water can

pep up

low vitality,

cleanse,

rebalance,

purify and relax.

Contrasting the energies of hot and cold water is an ancient practice that is still beneficial today. At spas, it is part of a total regime of treatments. At home, hydrotherapy means building on your normal bath and shower routine. To practise hydrotherapy both safely and effectively depends on the temperature of the water and what you add to it. Learn to use water in different ways and with different temperatures.

relaxing with water

Wake up to an energising cool shower or a cold sponge-down to strengthen your immune system, stimulate circulation and close pores. At the end of the day, soak in a hot ten-minute bath to induce perspiration, release toxins and alleviate tension.

Caution: if you are worried about any method or treatment suggested here, first check with your doctor.

different
temperatures
have a variety of
effects on your
effects on your
body. A whole
range is used
in hydrotherapy.

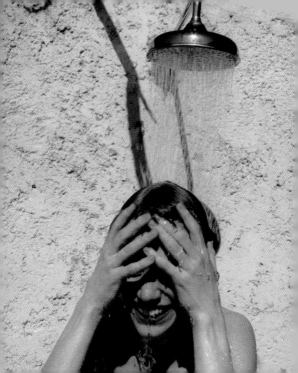

To tone skin, stimulate metabolism, help and improve your immune system. Only use if you are fit, with no blood pressure or heart problems. The cold can affect your heart rate and make your blood pressure rise slightly. Very cold? Enjoy for only a few seconds. Slightly warmer? Two minutes maximum.

Tepid: 29–36°C (85–97°F)

Similar to body temperature,

temperature ranges

tepid water is great for a bath-tub soak from 15 minutes to an hour, though your metabolism won't be stimulated sufficiently to expel many toxins.

Hot: 36–38°C (100–107°F)

Ideal for relieving muscle spasm, aches and pains, aiding detoxification and generally relaxing, it's best to take a hot bath – from five to fifteen min-utes maximum – at the end of the day when you can lie down afterwards or go to sleep.

Use a thermometer to check the temperature of the water. Do not run a hot bath and step straight into it. Get into a warm bath first then increase the temperature gradually by adding more hot water. Go easy with a cold bath, too. Avoid extreme temperatures on your skin. Plain baths or ones with salts, seaweed, hot and cold showers, essential oils and herbs, are all part of essential hydrotherapy.

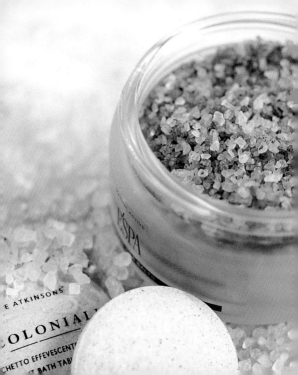

Invigorate skin while still dry with a five-minute skin-brushing session to sweep away dead cells, break down 'orange-peel' areas and to stimulate the lymph glands, the key to getting rid of waste matter. Use a natural bristle brush or loofah and long, gentle, sweeping strokes, working towards the heart. Follow with a warm shower or bath. Salt rubs improve circulation, helping to dispel as many toxins as possible. They also exfoliate, clearing the way so that bath additives can penetrate your skin more efficiently.

baths and rubs

Contrast sitz baths, are ones in which your bottom sits in hot water while your feet are placed in cold – then vice versa, helping to kick-start sluggish lymphatic system, and will detoxify and energise.

Detox baths, like Epsom Salt baths, are taken tepid or hot, to induce perspiration and detoxify the system. Top up gradually with hot water so you keep up a good sweat.

Thalassotherapy baths, or seaweed and seawater therapies, contain vitamins and minerals that can be absorbed through the skin to help firm and

tone, rebalance, detoxify, energise
and hydrate.

Oatmeal baths moisturise and gently
soften skin.

Herbal and essential oil baths soothe or
recharge and rebalance your system.

Caution: extremes in water temperature
and additives can have potential side-
effects, especially if you have high blood
pressure, heart disease, diabetes or if
you are pregnant. If in doubt, always
seek medical advice first.

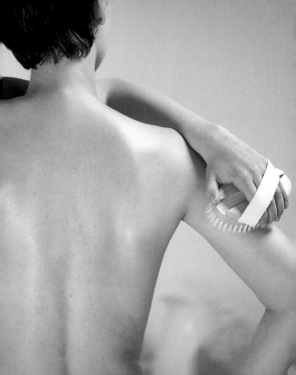

The Contrast Sitz Bath make sure your bathroom is warm. Use a plastic baby bath filled with cold water to fit into the foot end of your main bath. Sit in a hot-water bath, navel-level, while dipping your feet in the cold-water bowl, then vice versa – two minutes each way.

The Epsom Salt Bath add 450 g (1 lb) of Epsom salts to a hot bath. Soak for around 20 minutes. Towel dry and wrap up to keep the heat in. Relax for two hours. Drink plenty of water.

bath recipes

The Oatmeal Bath tie about 450 g (1 lb) of oatmeal in a piece of gauze. Hang it under the hot tap while the bath is running so that the flowing water carries all the moisturising ingredients with it. After about 20 minutes, step out of the bath and gently pat skin dry.

The Herbal Bath wrap up 50–100 g (2–4 oz) of dried herbs (try lavender, chamomile, marjoram and rosemary) in a muslin cloth, hang under running hot water. Then dip it in tepid bath water to infuse. Soak in your bath for 15–20 minutes.

The Seaweed Bath wrap a handful of dried seaweed in a muslin cloth. Hang it under the running hot water tap so the beneficial mineral salts, vitamins and trace elements flow into your bath. Soak in tepid water for 20 minutes.

Caution: take care if you're allergic to iodine.

The Salt Rub mix sea salt with water, or a body oil such as wheatgerm oil, to make sure the grains stick together. Rub briskly all over your body using circular movements in the direction of the heart. Rinse off under a warm shower. Rub oil over your skin. Rest or sleep.

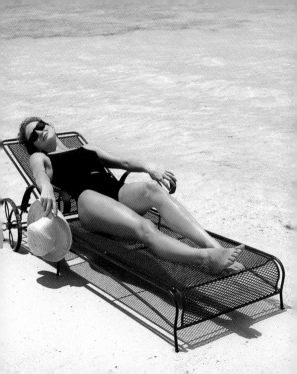

the therapeutic powers
of aromatherapy
– the science of
essential oils – is an
age-old practice with its
roots in
ancient Egypt.

aroma

therapy

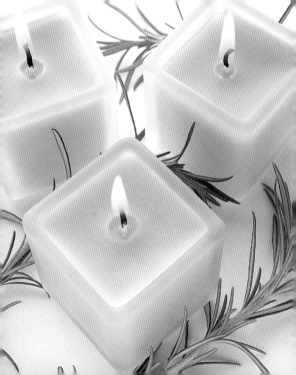

essential oils are highly
concentrated plant
substances used
to lift your mood
and relax
your mind.

33

Essential oils are absorbed through the skin and into the bloodstream. However, as pure extracted oils are highly concentrated, they should never be used directly on skin. To avoid skin irritation always dilute first in a carrier oil such as pure wheatgerm oil, nourishing grapeseed, softening apricot kernel or almond oil (baby oil or cooking oil is not suitable) or with a base lotion.

Seek professional advice from a trained aromatherapist and/or doctor before using essential oils if you suffer from skin allergies, epilepsy, high blood

using essential oils safely

pressure, are breastfeeding, pregnant, or have any other medical condition.

- Asthmatics should avoid directly inhaling pure essential oils – they could bring on an asthma attack.
- Keep oils away from eyes. If affected, wash eyes immediately with plenty of water. Seek medical advice.
- Do not take internally. Keep bottles out of reach of children. If swallowed, seek medical advice immediately.
- Pure essential oils are flammable.
- Avoid contact with plastic, polished or painted surfaces.

Chamomile: dissolves tension, induces sleep, skin-soothing.

Geranium: mood-lifting, good for depression. Helps relieve muscle ache and pre-menstrual fluid retention.

Grapefruit: tangy and revitalising, cleansing and purifying, helps detoxification. Relaxes muscles and relieves nervous tension.

Lavender: for a relaxed mood. An anti-septic, soothing oil. Avoid during the first three months of pregnancy.

Lemon grass: refreshing, uplifting, anti-septic. A powerful tonic.

10 oils and their benefits

Patchouli: calming and uplifting, relieves stress and anxiety. An anti-inflammatory and antiseptic used to treat skin disorders including acne and eczema.

Rose: stress-relieving, confidence-boosting and perfect if you're feeling vulnerable or tired with life. A restorative aroma for dry skin.

Rosemary: stimulating, invigorating and antiseptic. Helps to restore vitality, concentration and memory. Do not use if pregnant, suffer from epilepsy or have high blood pressure.

Sandalwood: reputed to be an aphrodisiac, a balancing oil with antiseptic properties that works well in massage and inhalations when you have a sore throat and dry cough.

Ylang Ylang: traditionally a love potion, it lulls you into a relaxed, harmonious state. Also skin toning.

Tip: all essential oils have an uplifting effect on your emotions. Follow your nose and invest in an oil with a smell you love – it could be telling you something.

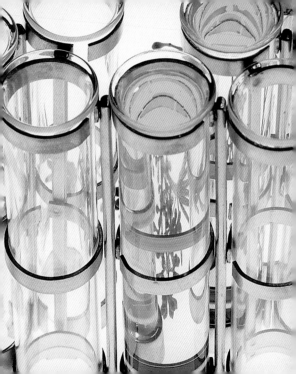

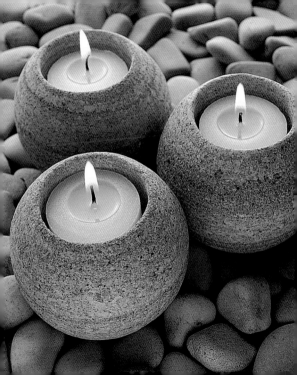

embark on a
sensory
journey
and surround
yourself with

aromas
that make you feel
at peace.

For the bath: add the recommended number of drops of essential oil (usually four to eight but no more than ten mixed with one tablespoon of vegetable oil like pure grapeseed. Pour under running warm bath water and agitate the water to disperse. The heat of the water releases the fragrance and helps the oils to be absorbed by the skin.

For a massage: mix up a total of 10–12 drops of one or more

essential oils in 2 tbsp of a carrier massage oil. Massage the area of your body that needs attention.

For a body lotion: add 5 drops of one or more essential oils to 2 tsp of a neutral lotion or cream base.

For a burner or vapouriser: add a little water to the dish and three to four drops of your chosen essential oil. Switch on the vapouriser or light the candle underneath. The warm

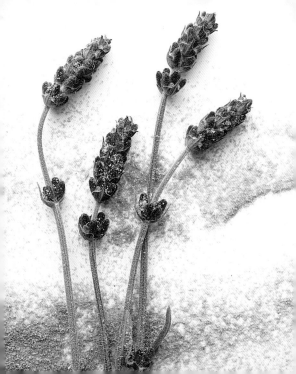

water helps the fragrance diffuse into the atmosphere.

For a facial moisturiser: put 2 drops of essential oil into 1 tsp of a neutral lotion or cream base. Avoid eyes.

Tip: start by using only one essence at a time to benefit from its impact. Then design your own blend or try out one of the recipes.

Dry-skin enricher for the face add 1½ tbsp jojoba oil to 2 drops rose oil, 3 drops sandalwood oil, 4 drops neroli oil, 3 drops patchouli oil. Gently massage over face.

A pick-me-up facial mask mix 1½ tbsp of apricot kernel oil with 4 drops sandalwood oil, 3 drops chamomile oil, 5 drops petitgrain oil. Massage onto face and leave for 10 minutes.

Body energiser mix 2 tbsp of almond oil with 2 drops rosemary oil, 4 drops grapefruit oil, 4 drops lime oil. Massage over body.

essential oil recipes

Cellulite Shifter mix 2 tbsp sweet almond oil with 2 drops lemon oil, 3 drops grapefruit oil, 3 drops juniper oil, 4 drops cypress oil. Massage over 'orange-peel' areas in circular movements, working in direction of heart.

Stress-reliever bath potion add 2 drops of lavender oil, 2 drops geranium oil, 1 drop rosewood to 4 tsp of carrier oil. Pour under hot running bath water. Relax for about 20 minutes otherwise the essential oils won't have time to work; any longer, and you'll feel too lethargic.

Wake-up-call bath potion add 2 drops bergamot, 2 drops lemon oil, 1 drop lemon grass oil to 4 tsp carrier oil. Pour under warm running bath water. Follow a 10-minute bath with a two-second cold shower to boost circulation and really wake you up!

48

Caution: one hour before applying a home-blended oil, do a patch test, particularly if you have sensitive skin.

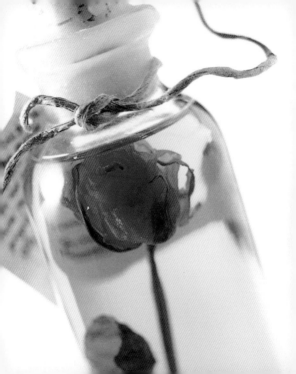

The power of touch should never be underestimated. Massage can relieve tense muscles, release nervous energy, boost circulation, help digestion, lower blood pressure and speed up the disposal of toxins. Even basic body stroking can calm and relieve any stiffness. Wear something loose and easy to move around in.

Effleurage, or skimming over: apply light pressure to the area you want to work on with moving hands, one hand following the other rhythmically, moving in a direction towards the heart.

massage moves

Single-point pressure: used in acupressure or shiatsu massage, firmly press on pain-relieving points with the fingers, thumbs or palms. Calms nerves or relieves problems like a headache.

Deep-muscle massage: for tense, aching muscles, make tiny circular movements with your finger or thumb which is pressed firmly into a muscle and then rotated. Always work in an upwards direction on the body.

Tapotement: to invigorate, tap with both hands alternately against the surface of the skin, with palms cupped.

'the way to good health is to have an aromatic bath and a scented massage every day'.

Hippocrates, 4th century BC

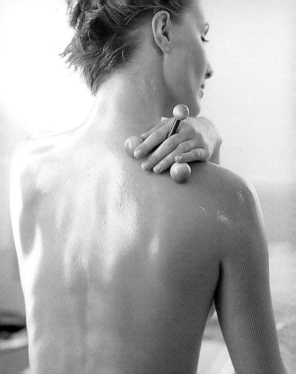

stretching and breathing
exercises will help you
unwind and relax.
They also play
a major part in the
self-cleansing
process.

switch

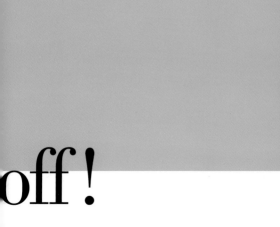

off !

Most of us use only half of our lung capacity. Relearning how to breathe with our diaphragm instead of upper chest will help our body's systems work in a healthier and more efficient way. Aim to move as much air in and out of your lungs as possible. Good breathing floods cells and tissues via the bloodstream with the oxygen they need to live and also efficiently removes carbon dioxide back into the air.

breathing

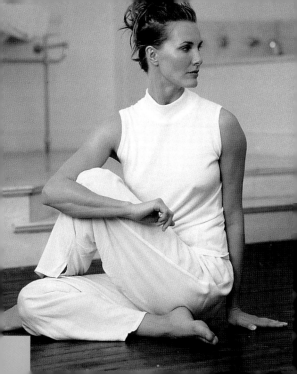

rest your hands on your rib-
cage at the side, just above
your waist. Breathe out completely. Now gently inhale
through the nose, letting your
abdomen swell as much as it
will to a slow count of five.
Continue breathing in through
your nose to another count of
five, this time letting your ribs
expand under your hands and
finally your chest. Make sure
you don't raise your shoulders

in the process. Hold your breath for a count of five. Now slowly and gently let it out through your mouth to the count of 10 noticing how your rib cage shrinks beneath your hands and pulling in with your abdomen until you have released all the air. Practise this exercise five times in a row, morning and evening.

Caution: if you feel dizzy, stop the exercise and relax.

Alternate nostril breathing: sitting comfortably, cross-legged on the floor or in a straight-backed chair, close your eyes and focus on your breathing, taking deep breaths in and out. Gently close your right nostril with your right thumb. Exhale through the left nostril to a count of four, then inhale through the left to a count of four. Release your right nostril and gently cover your left nostril with your little finger.

Exhale fully through the right nostril to a count of four. Inhale through the right to a count of four. Make sure your breathing is slow and steady and your neck and shoulders are relaxed. Repeat this sequence six to ten times. When exhaling empty your lungs completely.

Caution: any dizziness, open your eyes and rest for a while, breathing normally.

Have a good stretch. This increases the flow of blood to and from muscles, helping them to flex and relax. It also stimulates the lymph glands, encouraging the removal of toxins from the body. Many yoga positions combine deep stretches with gentle movement and slow rhythmic breathing. Warm up for a few minutes by walking around the room, swinging and circling your arms.

stretching

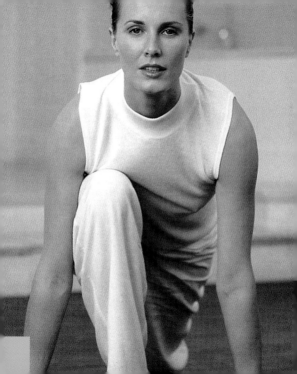

The upper body stretch: stand with feet parallel, hip-width apart. Bend knees slightly. Then bend forwards from the waist, linking hands together and stretching them away in front of you. Hold this position for 30 seconds, breathing deeply through your nose, not your mouth. Drop your heels to come up gently.

Tadasana or the Mountain posture: to lengthen your spine, align your body, help your breathing. Stand straight with feet parallel, hip-width apart. Knees relaxed but not bent. Gently inhale up through your body. As you exhale through your nose, drop your tailbone and pull lower abdominal muscles in gently. Aim to feel light, comfortable, with no tension in the shoulders.

Caution: do not stretch until it hurts. Slowly move out of the pose if you feel pain.

and combat stress with visualisation. Conjuring up in your mind images of happy places or events can stimulate your body's own healing powers.

66 Lie down in the yoga 'corpse' pose: on your back, arms out at about 45°, palms facing upwards, legs straight down. Check that your body is in alignment. Now close your eyes and mentally sweep through your body from top to

creative visualisation

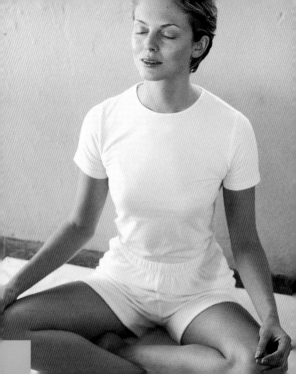

toe, relaxing tense muscles. Breathe slowly, gently, deeply, rhythmically.

Recall a place you really enjoyed being in, such as a beautiful white beach fringed with palm trees. See the clear blue sea stretching out to the horizon. Look up at the bright blue sky and enjoy the moment. Walk around enjoying the sounds, colours and smells. Feel the warmth of sand between your toes, the fresh sensation of sea water bathing your feet.

Repeat some positive affirmations to yourself to increase the feeling of peace and calm, for instance as 'I am feeling warm and relaxed … I am letting go of all stress … I am content with myself …' When you feel you are ready, bring yourself back to reality and enjoy a gentle stretch.

Mind and body workouts like yoga and t'ai chi will build up strength, co-ordination, flexibility and balance. They are also excellent stress-busting therapies.

Originating in China some 800 years ago, the aim of t'ai chi is to balance the emotional and physical energies of yin (cool, dark, negative energy) and yang (hot, light, positive energy) through slow, fluid controlled movements.

yoga and tai chi

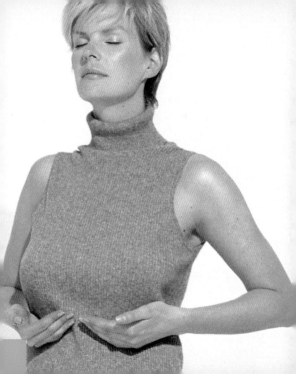

By meditating on these mea-
sured movements, in which you
flow with the direction of
energy, your mind is focused
away from whatever tension
you may be feeling.

Try this balancing chi exercise
to calm, relax and energise:
stand straight and still, feet
hip-width apart. Bring your
hands in towards your navel,
two inches in front, palms up
and fingers facing each other.
Now raise your hands to your

chest and rise up on your toes as you breathe in. Turn your palms downwards, drop your heels and let your hands sink down to your navel as you breathe out. Repeat slowly and rhythmically several times con-centrating on your breathing. When you start to feel warm your energy is balancing.

reach new energy levels
by spring cleaning
your body to give
your system
a rest.

spa

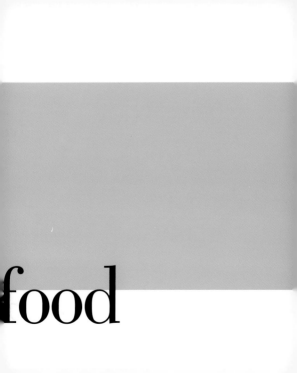

food

cleanse
your body
and you'll also
give your
immune system
a quick boost.

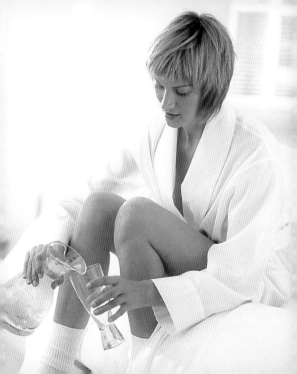

Drinking and eating nothing but fresh
fruit and/or vegetables on a one-day spa
detox is one of the best ways to start
breaking down a build-up of toxins at
cellular level.

Vegetables maintain, repair and build
up our body's tissues and cells.

Fruits are good cleansers and revitalisers
as well as a valuable source of vitamins,
minerals and amino acids.

The riper the fruit and vegetables
(preferably organic) the more vitamins
and minerals they will contain.

restoring your balance

- Fruit juices are high in natural sugars, so dilute each serving with water.
- Eat foods rich in vitamin A and folic acid, such as dark green or orange vegetables and orange juice.
- Eat iron-rich foods like peas, leafy green vegetables and dried beans.
- Stimulants like caffeine, chocolate, cigarettes and stress itself, are all energy-sappers. They may create energy in the short term, but long term, the effect is always bad.

'Yes' foods

Herbal teas and bottled or filtered water.

The best cleansing fruit juices are fresh apple, grape, grapefruit, lemon, lime, mango, melon, orange, papaya, peach, pear, pineapple, strawberry,

watermelon.

The best cleansing vegetable juices are fresh beetroot, carrot, celery, cucumber, spinach and watercress.

Steamed vegetables.

'yes' and 'no' food lists

'No' foods

- Refined foods like white pasta, white bread, white rice, sugar, biscuits, cakes, crisps and tinned or processed foods.
- Tea, coffee, alcohol, fizzy drinks.
- Dairy products, animal and vegetable fat.
- Food with added salt, salty snacks and foods like olives, pickles, sauces and stock cubes. These will raise your blood pressure.
- Dried fruit.

The ultimate natural body cleanser, water is the only fluid your body really needs. The body is made up of around 70% water – every chemical reaction that takes place relies on vital water power to be successful. Water helps to transport nutrients, regulates body temperature and is vital to the digestive process and the elimination of toxins. Drinking plenty of water will help stave off headaches, colds, flu, con-

nature's cleanser

stipation, cystitis, kidney stones and mood swings. Keeping your body hydrated can also reduce fluid retention and improve the texture and condition of your skin helping to prevent premature dry skin and wrinkles. Health experts agree that you should drink about eight glasses of water a day – more if it's hot, after exercising, or after a relaxing warm bath, which can leave you feeling dehydrated.

Keep a glass of water near you constantly. First thing in the morning, drink water to invigorate and cleanse. Have a small glass 10–15 minutes before each meal to metabolise nutrients and swell fibre. Mid-morning, mid-afternoon and early evening are low-energy times, so refresh with aqua power. At night, drink water to help you rest and regulate your body temperature. Different brands of mineral waters contain different levels of minerals such as magnesium, potassium, sodium, bone-building calcium and acidity-reducing bicarbonates. If you cannot get bottled natural mineral water from a guaranteed untainted source, it is best to filter it before drinkng or cooking with it. Still water is best though some mineral waters are naturally effervescent. Avoid artificially carbonated water. It depletes your minerals.

Juices are a healthy alternative to raw fruit and vegetables. They are ideal spring cleaners, giving your digestive system a much-needed rest. Their nutrient-rich, high-water content is released straight into your blood stream in just a few minutes, helping to boost the immune system and dispel toxins.

Home-made juices should be drunk immediately. They oxidise rapidly on contact with air and lose their vitamin C. Always dilute juices with still mineral water and drink up to 230 ml (8 fl oz) of juice during the day. Sprouted pulses like alfalfa or chickpeas, and seeds like sunflower and pumpkin, can be whizzed up in the blender too.

juice recipes

Pineapple and Apple

½ medium-sized pineapple • 3 apples

• 2 limes

Strawberry, Apple and Citrus Fruit

handful of strawberries • 1 orange

• 1 grapefruit • 2 apples

Papaya and Peach

½ papaya • ½ peach • 50 ml (2 fl oz) still

mineral water

Carrot and Celery

2 sticks celery • ½ lemon • 2 carrots

Peppers and Cucumber

¼ green (bell) pepper • ¼ red (bell) pepper
• ⅓ large cucumber

Fruit 'n' veg mix

3 carrots • 2 apples • 3 sticks celery • 2.5 mm
(1 in) root ginger

Juice each ingredient separately and, using a
spoon, blend.

Caution: avoid juices if you suffer from diabetes,
gastritis, obesity, kidney or heart disease, candida
or bowl disorder if you are underweight, breastfeeding or pregnant.

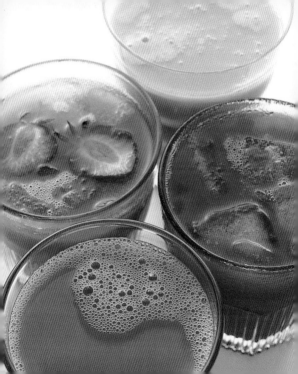

On rising – a cup of warm water with a squeeze of fresh lemon juice.

Breakfast – fresh whole fruits, fruit salad, fruit or vegetable juice.

Lunch – fresh whole fruit, juice drink or hot or cold meal option (given opposite). If you prefer, steam some vegetables.

Mid Afternoon – see Snack Attacks.

Dinner – fresh whole fruit, juice drink or hot or cold meal option or steamed vegetables.

Caution: follow for one day only. If you have any medical condition, seek professional advice first.

spa-day menu

Cold meal option – Raw vegetable salad

2 stalks celery • 3 oz (75 g) white cabbage

• 1 carrot • 2 spring onions • 1 green pepper

• ½ cucumber • 1 iceberg lettuce • 1 avocado

• 1 raw beetroot • 1 turnip

Slice or chop all the vegetables and place on

lettuce leaves.

Hot meal option – Energy-giving soup

4 carrots • ½ bunch broccoli • 3 celery stalks

1 onion • ½ bunch parsley • ½ lettuce

Peel and chop vegetables. Put in pan, cover with

water, bring to the boil. Leave to simmer for 30

minutes. Strain. For extra flavour, stir in Japanese

miso paste or organic stock, available from health food shops.

When hunger-pangs strike try some of these: sunflower and pumpkin seeds, crudités: red pepper, carrot, cucumber, cauliflower, raisins or delicious, nutritious sea vegetables such as wakame, kombu, dulse seaweeds, which are available from health food stores.

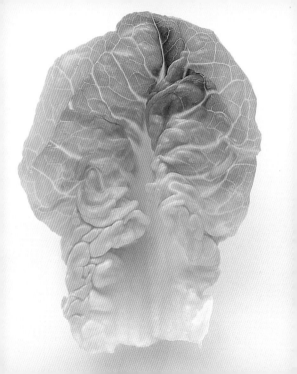

this is your chance to
shut the door on
the world, relax,
spoil and pamper
yourself.

spa envi

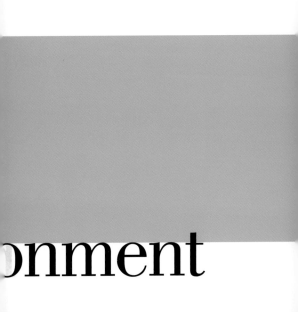

onment

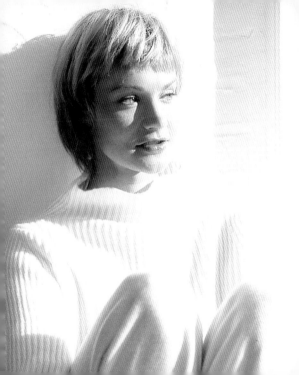

make advance
preparations: clear
your diary, tidy up 97
and invest
in spa essentials.

A light and airy space is a healthy environment. Wake up to a sunny light. If your bathroom has no natural daylight, put in a halogen rather than tungsten bulb for a fresh, white clean light. Relax with a low-level soft light. Transform the humble bath tub into a perfumed, candlelit haven. Make sure the rooms you'll be retreating to are warm. If your bathroom is cold, you will never attempt anything but a

preparations...

too-hot shower or bath and you won't be able to relax. A sufficiently ventilated bathroom will also leave you feeling calm and invigorated. Let the constant build-up of steam find an outlet so germs can't breed. In spas, bathrooms are designated 'wet' areas, changing rooms 'wet and dry' and relaxing rooms 'dry'.

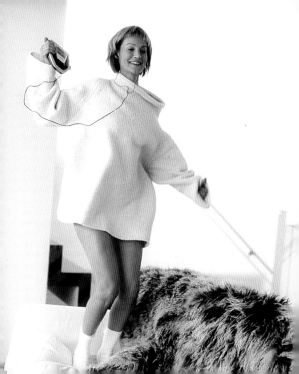

the more you rest and
exercise the better
the results.

101

All your energy
will be put
into healing.

Surround yourself with pure, aroma-uplifting air. An aroma candle or burner infused with soothing essences like lavender, rose and geranium, will create a heavenly atmosphere. Citrus scents like orange and lemon will uplift, while marine notes will remind you of sea breezes. Match the scent to the fragrance of the essential oils you are bathing in to intensify the therapeutic effect. Enjoy soothing sounds. Sound creates

breathe easy

privacy and a cassette or CD player in a room allows you to be in your own space. Drift away to the sounds of nature. New Age music tapes are perfect for the natural sounds of the sea, the call of dolphins, or age-old chants and mantras. Alternatively, listen to soothing classical music. In your rest periods, enjoy that book you've been meaning to read, or close your eyes and listen to a talking book on tape.

First invest in a few spa essentials. Then you're ready to create your own tranquil haven from the world.

Soft towelling robe • Cotton slippers • Fluffy towels • Long-bristled body brush • Sponge • Pure glycerine soap • Essential oils and carrier oil • Batteries for your cassette player • Soothing music tapes/CDs • Book or magazine • Mineral water • Sea Salt • Bath ingredients • Fresh and healthy snacks • Fruit and vegetables.

spa day checklist

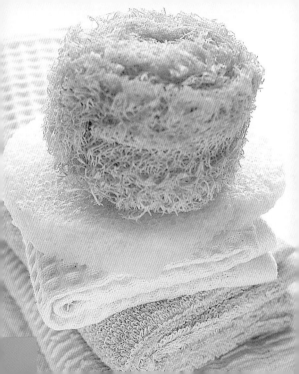

peace, quiet, serious
self-indulgence:
Do as little, or as much, as
you like.
This is your time
to relax and recharge.
Enjoy it.

your

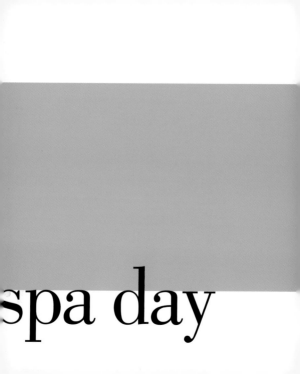

spa day

Drink throughout the day. Choose mineral or filter water and herb such as chamomile, lemon balm or rosehip for a soothing, cleansing effect.

morning

7.45 am Wake-up drink of cleansing, revitalising warm water with a squeeze of fresh lemon juice

8.00 am Breathing exercise: Yogic Energy Booster

8.45 am Cool shower or sponge-down or Contrast Sitz Bath

9.00 am Breakfast

the one-day spa

9.15 am Treatment: Body Brushing

9.45 am Treatment: Bath

10.00 am Rest and Relaxation

10.45 am Stretching Exercises

11.45 am Treatment: Massage followed
by Aromatherapy treatment

12.45 pm Lunch

afternoon

1.15 pm Rest and Relaxation

1.45 pm T'ai Chi Exercise

2.30 pm Rest. Surround yourself with
pure aromas

3.00 pm Creative Visualisation

4.00 pm Salt Rub

5.00 pm Rest and Relaxation

6.00 pm Breathing Exercises

7.00 pm Supper

7.15 pm Rest and Relaxation

8.00 pm Relaxing Aromatherapy Bath

And so to bed ... ready to face the next day calmer, more revitalised, more able to cope with life's challenges.

Sleep well.

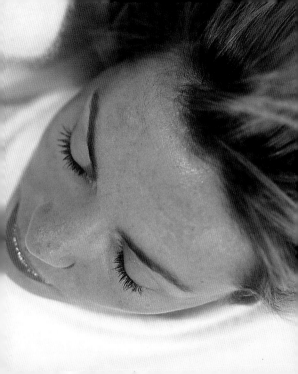

First published in 2000 by
HarperCollins*Illustrated*
An imprint of HarperCollins*Publishers*
77–85 Fulham Palace Road
London W6 8JB

The HarperCollins website address is: www.**fire**and**water**.com

Published in association with The National Magazine Company Limited.
Good Housekeeping is a registered trademark of The National Magazine Company
Limited and the Hearst Corporation.

The Good Housekeeping website address is www.goodhousekeeping.co.uk

British Library Cataloguing-in-Publication Data
A catalogue record for this book is available from the British Library.
ISBN 0-00-710446-4

Colour reproduction by Colourscan, Singapore
Printed and bound in China by Imago